10·7·11   56688   18.05
BT

D1026963

Global strategy to reduce the harmful use of alcohol

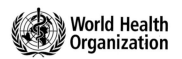

WHO Library Cataloguing-in-Publication Data

Global strategy to reduce the harmful use of alcohol.

1.Alcohol drinking - adverse effects. 2.Social control - methods. 3.Alcoholism - prevention and control. 4.Public policy. I.World Health Organization.

ISBN 978 92 4 159993 1   (NLM classification: WM 274)

© **World Health Organization 2010**

All rights reserved. Publications of the World Health Organization can be obtained from WHO Press, World Health Organization, 20 Avenue Appia, 1211 Geneva 27, Switzerland (tel.: +41 22 791 3264; fax: +41 22 791 4857; e-mail: bookorders@who.int). Requests for permission to reproduce or translate WHO publications – whether for sale or for noncommercial distribution – should be addressed to WHO Press, at the above address (fax: +41 22 791 4806; e-mail: permissions@who.int).

The designations employed and the presentation of the material in this publication do not imply the expression of any opinion whatsoever on the part of the World Health Organization concerning the legal status of any country, territory, city or area or of its authorities, or concerning the delimitation of its frontiers or boundaries. Dotted lines on maps represent approximate border lines for which there may not yet be full agreement.

The mention of specific companies or of certain manufacturers' products does not imply that they are endorsed or recommended by the World Health Organization in preference to others of a similar nature that are not mentioned. Errors and omissions excepted, the names of proprietary products are distinguished by initial capital letters.

All reasonable precautions have been taken by the World Health Organization to verify the information contained in this publication. However, the published material is being distributed without warranty of any kind, either expressed or implied. The responsibility for the interpretation and use of the material lies with the reader. In no event shall the World Health Organization be liable for damages arising from its use.

Design and layout: L'IV Com Sàrl, Le Mont-sur-Lausanne, Switzerland.

Printed in Italy.

TABLE OF CONTENTS

FOREWORD

The harmful use of alcohol causes an estimated 2.5 million deaths every year, of which a significant proportion occur in the young. Alcohol use is the third leading risk factor for poor health globally. A wide variety of alcohol-related problems can have devastating impacts on individuals and their families and can seriously affect community life. The harmful use of alcohol is one of the four most common modifiable and preventable risk factors for major noncommunicable diseases (NCDs). There is also emerging evidence that the harmful use of alcohol contributes to the health burden caused by communicable diseases such as, for example, tuberculosis and HIV/AIDS.

Reducing the harmful use of alcohol by effective policy measures and by providing a relevant infrastructure to successfully implement those measures is much more than a public health issue. Indeed, it is a development issue, since the level of risk associated with the harmful use of alcohol in developing countries is much higher than that in high-income countries where people are increasingly protected by comprehensive laws and interventions – and by mechanisms to ensure that these are implemented.

The global strategy to reduce the harmful use of alcohol, endorsed by the Sixty-third World Health Assembly in May 2010, recognizes the close links between the harmful use of alcohol and socioeconomic development. It represents the commitment by the Member States of the World Health Organization to sustained action at all levels. It also builds on several WHO global and regional strategic initiatives, including the action plan for the global strategy for the prevention and control of noncommunicable diseases which was endorsed by the World Health Assembly in 2008.

Indeed, WHO is witnessing how public health policy-makers in developing countries and economies in transition are increasingly challenged to formulate effective strategies to address the public health problems caused by the harmful use of alcohol. Workable solutions exist and the global strategy provides a portfolio of policy options and interventions that should be considered for implementation in each country as integral parts of national policy, as well as within broader development frameworks. The global strategy also sets priority areas for global action that is intended to promote, support and complement relevant actions at local, national and regional levels. Honouring the spirit of the Paris Declaration on Aid Effectiveness, WHO calls on international development partners to respond favourably to requests from developing countries for technical support in implementing and adapting these policy options according to national priorities and contexts.

The consensus reached on the global strategy and its endorsement by the World Health Assembly is the outcome of close collaboration between WHO Member States and the WHO secretariat. The process that led to the development of the global strategy included consultations with other stakeholders, such as civil society groups and economic operators. Similarly, the implementation of the global strategy will require active collaboration with Member States, with appropriate engagement of international development partners, civil society, the private sector, as well as public health and research institutions. As we move forward, WHO will continue to involve relevant stakeholders in efforts to achieve the strategy goals and objectives.

I am confident that by working together towards the objectives of the global strategy, we can reduce the negative health and social consequences of the harmful use of alcohol and make our communities healthier, safer and more pleasant places in which to live, work and spend our leisure time.

Dr Ala Alwan
Assistant Director-General
Noncommunicable Diseases and Mental Health
World Health Organization

THE GLOBAL STRATEGY TO REDUCE THE HARMFUL USE OF ALCOHOL[1]

Setting the scene

1. The harmful use of alcohol[2] has a serious effect on public health and is considered to be one of the main risk factors for poor health globally. In the context of this draft strategy, the concept of the harmful use of alcohol[3] is broad and encompasses the drinking that causes detrimental health and social consequences for the drinker, the people around the drinker and society at large, as well as the patterns of drinking that are associated with increased risk of adverse health outcomes. The harmful use of alcohol compromises both individual and social development. It can ruin the lives of individuals, devastate families, and damage the fabric of communities.

2. The harmful use of alcohol is a significant contributor to the global burden of disease and is listed as the third leading risk factor for premature deaths and disabilities in the world.[4] It is estimated that 2.5 million people worldwide died of alcohol-related causes in 2004, including 320 000 young people between 15 and 29 years of age. Harmful use of alcohol was responsible for 3.8% of all deaths in the world in 2004 and 4.5% of the global burden of disease as measured in disability-adjusted life years lost, even when consideration is given to the modest protective effects, especially on coronary heart disease, of low consumption of alcohol for some people aged 40 years or older.

3. Harmful drinking is a major avoidable risk factor for neuropsychiatric disorders and other noncommunicable diseases such as cardiovascular diseases, cirrhosis of the liver and various cancers. For some diseases there is no evidence of a threshold effect in the relationship between the risk and level of alcohol consumption. The harmful use of alcohol is also associated with several infectious diseases like HIV/AIDS, tuberculosis and pneumonia. A significant proportion of the disease burden attributable to harmful drinking arises from unintentional and intentional injuries, including those due to road traffic crashes and violence, and suicides. Fatal injuries attributable to alcohol consumption tend to occur in relatively young people.

4. The degree of risk for harmful use of alcohol varies with age, sex and other biological characteristics of the consumer as well as with the setting and context in which the drinking takes place. Some vulnerable or at-risk groups and individuals have increased

---

1 See resolution WHA63.13 (page 27).

2 An alcoholic beverage is a liquid that contains ethanol (ethyl alcohol, commonly called "alcohol") and is intended for drinking. In most countries with a legal definition of "alcoholic beverage" a threshold for content of ethanol by volume in a beverage is set at ≥ 0.5% or 1.0%. The predominant categories of alcoholic beverages are beers, wines and spirits.

3 The word "harmful" in this strategy refers only to public-health effects of alcohol consumption, without prejudice to religious beliefs and cultural norms in any way.

4 See document A60/14 Add.1 for a global assessment of public-health problems caused by harmful use of alcohol, and *Global Health Risks: Mortality and burden of disease attributable to selected major risk factors.* Geneva, World Health Organization, 2009.

susceptibility to the toxic, psychoactive and dependence-producing properties of ethanol. At the same time low risk patterns of alcohol consumption at the individual level may not be associated with occurrence or significantly increased probability of negative health and social consequences.

5. A substantial scientific knowledge base exists for policy-makers on the effectiveness and cost-effectiveness of strategies and interventions to prevent and reduce alcohol-related harm.[1] Although much of the evidence comes from high-income countries, the results of meta-analyses and reviews of the available evidence[2] provide sufficient knowledge to inform policy recommendations in terms of comparative effectiveness and cost-effectiveness of selected policy measures. With better awareness, there are increased responses at national, regional and global levels. However, these policy responses are often fragmented and do not always correspond to the magnitude of the impact on health and social development.

Challenges and opportunities

6. The present commitment to reducing the harmful use of alcohol provides a great opportunity for improving health and social well-being and for reducing the existing alcohol-attributable disease burden. However, there are considerable challenges that have to be taken into account in global or national initiatives or programmes. These include the following:

(a) **Increasing global action and international cooperation.** The current relevant health, cultural and market trends worldwide mean that harmful use of alcohol will continue to be a global health issue. These trends should be recognized and appropriate responses implemented at all levels. In this respect, there is a need for global guidance and increased international collaboration to support and complement regional and national actions.

(b) **Ensuring intersectoral action.** The diversity of alcohol-related problems and measures necessary to reduce alcohol-related harm points to the need for comprehensive action across numerous sectors. Policies to reduce the harmful use of alcohol must reach beyond the health sector, and appropriately engage such sectors as development, transport, justice, social welfare, fiscal policy, trade, agriculture, consumer policy, education and employment, as well as civil society and economic operators.

(c) **According appropriate attention.** Preventing and reducing harmful use of alcohol is often given a low priority among decision-makers despite compelling evidence of its serious public health effects. In addition, there is a clear discrepancy between the increasing availability and affordability of alcohol beverages in many developing and low- and middle-income countries and those countries' capability and capacity to meet the additional public health burden that follows. Unless this problem is given the attention it deserves, the spread of harmful drinking practices and norms will continue.

---

1 See document A60/14 for evidence-based strategies and interventions to reduce alcohol-related harm.

2 See, for example: WHO Technical Report Series, No. 944, 2007 and *Evidence for the effectiveness and cost-effectiveness of interventions to reduce alcohol-related harm.* Copenhagen, World Health Organization Regional Office for Europe, 2009.

(d) **Balancing different interests.** Production, distribution, marketing and sales of alcohol create employment and generate considerable income for economic operators and tax revenue for governments at different levels. Public health measures to reduce harmful use of alcohol are sometimes judged to be in conflict with other goals like free markets and consumer choice and can be seen as harming economic interests and reducing government revenues. Policy-makers face the challenge of giving an appropriate priority to the promotion and protection of population health while taking into account other goals, obligations, including international legal obligations, and interests. It should be noted in this respect that international trade agreements generally recognize the right of countries to take measures to protect human health, provided that these are not applied in a manner which would constitute a means of unjustifiable or arbitrary discrimination or disguised restrictions to trade. In this regard, national, regional and international efforts should take into account the impact of harmful use of alcohol.

(e) **Focusing on equity.** Population-wide rates of drinking of alcoholic beverages are markedly lower in poorer societies than in wealthier ones. However, for a given amount of consumption, poorer populations may experience disproportionately higher levels of alcohol-attributable harm. There is a great need to develop and implement effective policies and programmes that reduce such social disparities both inside a country and between countries. Such policies are also needed in order to generate and disseminate new knowledge about the complex relationship between harmful consumption of alcohol and social and health inequity, particularly among indigenous populations, minority or marginalized groups and in developing countries.

(f) **Considering the "context" in recommending actions.** Much of the published evidence of effectiveness of alcohol-related policy interventions comes from high-income countries, and concerns have been expressed that their effectiveness depends on context and may not be transferrable to other settings. However, many interventions to reduce harmful use of alcohol have been implemented in a wide variety of cultures and settings, and their results are often consistent and in line with the underpinning theories and evidence base accumulated in other similar public health areas. The focus for those developing and implementing policies should be on appropriate tailoring of effective interventions to accommodate local contexts and on appropriate monitoring and evaluation to provide feedback for further action.

(g) **Strengthening information.** Systems for collecting, analysing and disseminating data on alcohol consumption, alcohol-related harm and policy responses have been developed by Member States, the WHO Secretariat, and some other stakeholders. There are still substantial gaps in knowledge and it is important to sharpen the focus on information and knowledge production and dissemination for further developments in this area, especially in developing and low- and middle-income countries. The WHO Global Information System on Alcohol and Health and integrated regional information systems provide the means to monitor better progress made in reducing harmful use of alcohol at the global and regional levels.

Aims and objectives

7. National and local efforts can produce better results when they are supported by regional and global action within agreed policy frames. Thus the purpose of the global strategy is to support and complement public health policies in Member States.

8. The vision behind the global strategy is improved health and social outcomes for individuals, families and communities, with considerably reduced morbidity and mortality due to harmful use of alcohol and their ensuing social consequences. It is envisaged that the global strategy will promote and support local, regional and global actions to prevent and reduce the harmful use of alcohol.

9. The global strategy aims to give guidance for action at all levels; to set priority areas for global action; and to recommend a portfolio of policy options and measures that could be considered for implementation and adjusted as appropriate at the national level, taking into account national circumstances, such as religious and cultural contexts, national public health priorities, as well as resources, capacities and capabilities.

10. The strategy has five objectives:

   (a) raised global awareness of the magnitude and nature of the health, social and economic problems caused by harmful use of alcohol, and increased commitment by governments to act to address the harmful use of alcohol;

   (b) strengthened knowledge base on the magnitude and determinants of alcohol-related harm and on effective interventions to reduce and prevent such harm;

   (c) increased technical support to, and enhanced capacity of, Member States for preventing the harmful use of alcohol and managing alcohol-use disorders and associated health conditions;

   (d) strengthened partnerships and better coordination among stakeholders and increased mobilization of resources required for appropriate and concerted action to prevent the harmful use of alcohol;

   (e) improved systems for monitoring and surveillance at different levels, and more effective dissemination and application of information for advocacy, policy development and evaluation purposes.

11. The harmful use of alcohol and its related public health problems are influenced by the general level of alcohol consumption in a population, drinking patterns and local contexts. Achieving the five objectives will require global, regional and national actions on the levels, patterns and contexts of alcohol consumption and the wider social determinants of health. Special attention needs to be given to reducing harm to people other than the drinker and to populations that are at particular risk from harmful use of alcohol, such as children, adolescents, women of child-bearing age, pregnant and breastfeeding women, indigenous peoples and other minority groups or groups with low socioeconomic status.

Guiding principles

12. The protection of the health of the population by preventing and reducing the harmful use of alcohol is a public health priority. The following principles will guide the development and implementation of policies at all levels; they reflect the multifaceted determinants of alcohol-related harm and the concerted multisectoral actions required to implement effective interventions.

(a) Public policies and interventions to prevent and reduce alcohol-related harm should be guided and formulated by public health interests and based on clear public health goals and the best available evidence.

(b) Policies should be equitable and sensitive to national, religious and cultural contexts.

(c) All involved parties have the responsibility to act in ways that do not undermine the implementation of public policies and interventions to prevent and reduce harmful use of alcohol.

(d) Public health should be given proper deference in relation to competing interests and approaches that support that direction should be promoted.

(e) Protection of populations at high risk of alcohol-attributable harm and those exposed to the effects of harmful drinking by others should be an integral part of policies addressing the harmful use of alcohol.

(f) Individuals and families affected by the harmful use of alcohol should have access to affordable and effective prevention and care services.

(g) Children, teenagers and adults who choose not to drink alcohol beverages have the right to be supported in their non-drinking behaviour and protected from pressures to drink.

(h) Public policies and interventions to prevent and reduce alcohol-related harm should encompass all alcoholic beverages and surrogate alcohol.[1]

National policies and measures

13. The harmful use of alcohol can be reduced if effective actions are taken by countries to protect their populations. Member States have a primary responsibility for formulating, implementing, monitoring and evaluating public policies to reduce the harmful use of alcohol. Such policies require a wide range of public health-oriented strategies for prevention and treatment. All countries will benefit from having a national strategy and appropriate legal frameworks to reduce harmful use of alcohol, regardless of the level of resources in the country. Depending on the characteristics of policy options and national circumstances, some policy options can be implemented by non-legal frameworks such as guidelines or voluntary restraints. Successful implementation of

---

1 In this strategy "surrogate alcohol" refers to liquids usually containing ethanol and not intended for consumption as beverages, that are consumed orally as substitutes for alcoholic beverages with the objective to producing intoxication or other effects associated with alcohol consumption.

measures should be assisted by monitoring impact and compliance and establishing and imposing sanctions for non-compliance with adopted laws and regulations.

14. Sustained political commitment, effective coordination, sustainable funding and appropriate engagement of subnational governments as well as from civil society and economic operators are essential for success. Many relevant decision-making authorities should be involved in the formulation and implementation of alcohol policies, such as health ministries, transportation authorities or taxation agencies. Governments need to establish effective and permanent coordination machinery, such as a national alcohol council, comprising senior representatives of many ministries and other partners, in order to ensure a coherent approach to alcohol policies and a proper balance between policy goals in relation to harmful use of alcohol and other public policy goals.

15. Health ministries have a crucial role in bringing together the other ministries and stakeholders needed for effective policy design and implementation. They should also ensure that planning and provision of prevention and treatment strategies and interventions are coordinated with those for other related health conditions with high public health priority such as illicit drug use, mental illness, violence and injuries, cardiovascular diseases, cancer, tuberculosis and HIV/AIDS.

16. The policy options and interventions available for national action can be grouped into 10 recommended target areas, which should be seen as supportive and complementary to each other. These 10 areas are:

(a) leadership, awareness and commitment

(b) health services' response

(c) community action

(d) drink-driving policies and countermeasures

(e) availability of alcohol

(f) marketing of alcoholic beverages

(g) pricing policies

(h) reducing the negative consequences of drinking and alcohol intoxication

(i) reducing the public health impact of illicit alcohol and informally produced alcohol[1]

(j) monitoring and surveillance.

17. The policy options and interventions proposed below for consideration by Member States for each of the 10 recommended target areas are based on current scientific knowledge, available evidence on effectiveness and cost-effectiveness, experience and good practices. Not all the policy options and interventions will be applicable

---

1 **Informally produced alcohol** means alcoholic beverages produced at home or locally by fermentation and distillation of fruits, grains, vegetables and the like, and often within the context of local cultural practices and traditions. Examples of informally produced alcoholic beverages include sorghum beer, palm wine and spirits produced from sugarcane, grains or other commodities.

or relevant for all Member States and some may be beyond available resources. As such, the measures should be implemented at the discretion of each Member State depending on national, religious and cultural contexts, national public health priorities, and available resources, and in accordance with constitutional principles and international legal obligations. Policy measures and interventions at the national level will be supported and complemented by global and regional efforts to reduce the harmful use of alcohol.

Policy options and interventions

Area 1. Leadership, awareness and commitment

18. Sustainable action requires strong leadership and a solid base of awareness and political will and commitment. The commitments should ideally be expressed through adequately funded comprehensive and intersectoral national policies that clarify the contributions, and division of responsibility, of the different partners involved. The policies must be based on available evidence and tailored to local circumstances, with clear objectives, strategies and targets. The policy should be accompanied by a specific action plan and supported by effective and sustainable implementation and evaluation mechanisms. The appropriate engagement of civil society and economic operators is essential.

19. For this area **policy options and interventions** include:

(a) developing or strengthening existing, comprehensive national and subnational strategies, plans of action and activities to reduce the harmful use of alcohol;

(b) establishing or appointing a main institution or agency, as appropriate, to be responsible for following up national policies, strategies and plans;

(c) coordinating alcohol strategies with work in other relevant sectors, including cooperation between different levels of governments, and with other relevant health-sector strategies and plans;

(d) ensuring broad access to information and effective education and public awareness programmes among all levels of society about the full range of alcohol-related harm experienced in the country and the need for, and existence of, effective preventive measures;

(e) raising awareness of harm to others and among vulnerable groups caused by drinking, avoiding stigmatization and actively discouraging discrimination against affected groups and individuals.

Area 2. Health services' response

20. Health services are central to tackling harm at the individual level among those with alcohol-use disorders and other health conditions caused by harmful use of alcohol. Health services should provide prevention and treatment interventions to individuals and families at risk of, or affected by, alcohol-use disorders and associated conditions. Another important role of health services and health professionals is to inform societies about the public health and social consequences of harmful use of alcohol, support communities in their efforts to reduce the harmful use of alcohol, and to advocate effective societal responses. Health services should reach out to, mobilize and involve a broad range of players outside the health sector. Health services response should be sufficiently strengthened and funded in a way that is commensurate with the magnitude of the public health problems caused by harmful use of alcohol.

21. For this area **policy options and interventions** include:

   (a) increasing capacity of health and social welfare systems to deliver prevention, treatment and care for alcohol-use and alcohol-induced disorders and co-morbid conditions, including support and treatment for affected families and support for mutual help or self-help activities and programmes;

   (b) supporting initiatives for screening and brief interventions for hazardous and harmful drinking at primary health care and other settings; such initiatives should include early identification and management of harmful drinking among pregnant women and women of child-bearing age;

   (c) improving capacity for prevention of, identification of, and interventions for individuals and families living with fetal alcohol syndrome and a spectrum of associated disorders;

   (d) development and effective coordination of integrated and/or linked prevention, treatment and care strategies and services for alcohol-use disorders and co-morbid conditions, including drug-use disorders, depression, suicides, HIV/AIDS and tuberculosis;

   (e) securing universal access to health including through enhancing availability, accessibility and affordability of treatment services for groups of low socioeconomic status;

   (f) establishing and maintaining a system of registration and monitoring of alcohol-attributable morbidity and mortality, with regular reporting mechanisms;

   (g) provision of culturally sensitive health and social services as appropriate.

Area 3. Community action

22. The impact of harmful use of alcohol on communities can trigger and foster local initiatives and solutions to local problems. Communities can be supported and empowered by governments and other stakeholders to use their local knowledge and expertise in adopting effective approaches to prevent and reduce the harmful use of alcohol by changing collective rather than individual behaviour while being sensitive to cultural norms, beliefs and value systems.

23. For this area **policy options and interventions** include:

   (a) supporting rapid assessments in order to identify gaps and priority areas for interventions at the community level;

(b) facilitating increased recognition of alcohol-related harm at the local level and promoting appropriate effective and cost-effective responses to the local determinants of harmful use of alcohol and related problems;

(c) strengthening capacity of local authorities to encourage and coordinate concerted community action by supporting and promoting the development of municipal policies to reduce harmful use of alcohol, as well as their capacity to enhance partnerships and networks of community institutions and nongovernmental organizations;

(d) providing information about effective community-based interventions, and building capacity at community level for their implementation;

(e) mobilizing communities to prevent the selling of alcohol to, and consumption of alcohol by, under-age drinkers, and to develop and support alcohol-free environments, especially for youth and other at-risk groups;

(f) providing community care and support for affected individuals and their families;

(g) developing or supporting community programmes and policies for subpopulations at particular risk, such as young people, unemployed persons and indigenous populations, specific issues like the production and distribution of illicit or informal-alcohol beverages and events at community level such as sporting events and town festivals.

Area 4. Drink-driving policies and countermeasures

24. Driving under the influence of alcohol seriously affects a person's judgment, coordination and other motor functions. Alcohol-impaired driving is a significant public health problem that affects both the drinker and in many cases innocent parties. Strong evidence-based interventions exist for reducing drink-driving. Strategies to reduce harm associated with drink-driving should include deterrent measures that aim to reduce the likelihood that a person will drive under the influence of alcohol, and measures that create a safer driving environment in order to reduce both the likelihood and severity of harm associated with alcohol-influenced crashes.

25. In some countries, the number of traffic-related injuries involving intoxicated pedestrians is substantial and should be a high priority for intervention.

26. For this area **policy options and interventions** include:

(a) introducing and enforcing an upper limit for blood alcohol concentration, with a reduced limit for professional drivers and young or novice drivers;

(b) promoting sobriety check points and random breath-testing;

(c) administrative suspension of driving licences;

(d) graduated licensing for novice drivers with zero-tolerance for drink-driving;

(e) using an ignition interlock, in specific contexts where affordable, to reduce drink-driving incidents;

(f)   mandatory driver-education, counselling and, as appropriate, treatment programmes;

(g)   encouraging provision of alternative transportation, including public transport until after the closing time for drinking places;

(h)   conducting public awareness and information campaigns in support of policy and in order to increase the general deterrence effect;

(i)   running carefully planned, high-intensity, well-executed mass media campaigns targeted at specific situations, such as holiday seasons, or audiences such as young people.

Area 5. Availability of alcohol

27. Public health strategies that seek to regulate the commercial or public availability of alcohol through laws, policies, and programmes are important ways to reduce the general level of harmful use of alcohol. Such strategies provide essential measures to prevent easy access to alcohol by vulnerable and high-risk groups. Commercial and public availability of alcohol can have a reciprocal influence on the social availability of alcohol and thus contribute to changing social and cultural norms that promotes harmful use of alcohol. The level of regulation on the availability of alcohol will depend on local circumstances, including social, cultural and economic contexts as well as existing binding international obligations. In some developing and low- and middle-income countries, informal markets are the main source of alcohol and formal controls on sale need to be complemented by actions addressing illicit or informally produced alcohol. Furthermore, restrictions on availability that are too strict may promote the development of a parallel illicit market. Secondary supply of alcohol, for example from parents or friends, needs also to be taken into consideration in measures on the availability of alcohol.

28. For this area **policy options and interventions** include:

(a)   establishing, operating and enforcing an appropriate system to regulate production, wholesaling and serving of alcoholic beverages that places reasonable limitations on the distribution of alcohol and the operation of alcohol outlets in accordance with cultural norms, by the following possible measures:

    (i)   introducing, where appropriate, a licensing system on retail sales, or public health oriented government monopolies;

    (ii)   regulating the number and location of on-premise and off-premise alcohol outlets;

    (iii) regulating days and hours of retail sales;

    (iv) regulating modes of retail sales of alcohol;

    (v)   regulating retail sales in certain places or during special events;

(b) establishing an appropriate minimum age for purchase or consumption of alcoholic beverages and other policies in order to raise barriers against sales to, and consumption of alcoholic beverages by, adolescents;

(c) adopting policies to prevent sales to intoxicated persons and those below the legal age and considering the introduction of mechanisms for placing liability on sellers and servers in accordance with national legislations;

(d) setting policies regarding drinking in public places or at official public agencies' activities and functions;

(e) adopting policies to reduce and eliminate availability of illicit production, sale and distribution of alcoholic beverages as well as to regulate or control informal alcohol.

Area 6. Marketing[1] of alcoholic beverages

29. Reducing the impact of marketing, particularly on young people and adolescents, is an important consideration in reducing harmful use of alcohol. Alcohol is marketed through increasingly sophisticated advertising and promotion techniques, including linking alcohol brands to sports and cultural activities, sponsorships and product placements, and new marketing techniques such as e-mails, SMS and podcasting, social media and other communication techniques. The transmission of alcohol marketing messages across national borders and jurisdictions on channels such as satellite television and the Internet, and sponsorship of sports and cultural events is emerging as a serious concern in some countries.

30. It is very difficult to target young adult consumers without exposing cohorts of adolescents under the legal age to the same marketing. The exposure of children and young people to appealing marketing is of particular concern, as is the targeting of new markets in developing and low- and middle-income countries with a current low prevalence of alcohol consumption or high abstinence rates. Both the content of alcohol marketing and the amount of exposure of young people to that marketing are crucial issues. A precautionary approach to protecting young people against these marketing techniques should be considered.

31. For this area **policy options and interventions** include:

(a) setting up regulatory or co-regulatory frameworks, preferably with a legislative basis, and supported when appropriate by self-regulatory measures, for alcohol marketing by:

(i) regulating the content and the volume of marketing;

(ii) regulating direct or indirect marketing in certain or all media;

(iii) regulating sponsorship activities that promote alcoholic beverages;

---

1 Marketing could refer, as appropriate and in accordance with national legislation, to any form of commercial communication or message that is designed to increase, or has the effect of increasing, the recognition, appeal and/or consumption of particular products and services. It could comprise anything that acts to advertise or otherwise promote a product or service.

(iv) restricting or banning promotions in connection with activities targeting young people;

(v) regulating new forms of alcohol marketing techniques, for instance social media;

(b) development by public agencies or independent bodies of effective systems of surveillance of marketing of alcohol products;

(c) setting up effective administrative and deterrence systems for infringements on marketing restrictions.

Area 7. Pricing policies

32. Consumers, including heavy drinkers and young people, are sensitive to changes in the price of drinks. Pricing policies can be used to reduce underage drinking, to halt progression towards drinking large volumes of alcohol and/or episodes of heavy drinking, and to influence consumers' preferences. Increasing the price of alcoholic beverages is one of the most effective interventions to reduce harmful use of alcohol. A key factor for the success of price-related policies in reducing harmful use of alcohol is an effective and efficient system for taxation matched by adequate tax collection and enforcement.

33. Factors such as consumer preferences and choice, changes in income, alternative sources for alcohol in the country or in neighbouring countries, and the presence or absence of other alcohol policy measures may influence the effectiveness of this policy option. Demand for different beverages may be affected differently. Tax increases can have different impacts on sales, depending on how they affect the price to the consumer. The existence of a substantial illicit market for alcohol complicates policy considerations on taxation in many countries. In such circumstances tax changes must be accompanied by efforts to bring the illicit and informal markets under effective government control. Increased taxation can also meet resistance from consumer groups and economic operators, and taxation policy will benefit from the support of information and awareness-building measures to counter such resistance.

34. For this area policy options and interventions include:

(a) establishing a system for specific domestic taxation on alcohol accompanied by an effective enforcement system, which may take into account, as appropriate, the alcoholic content of the beverage;

(b) regularly reviewing prices in relation to level of inflation and income;

(c) banning or restricting the use of direct and indirect price promotions, discount sales, sales below cost and flat rates for unlimited drinking or other types of volume sales;

(d) establishing minimum prices for alcohol where applicable;

(e) providing price incentives for non-alcoholic beverages;

(f) reducing or stopping subsidies to economic operators in the area of alcohol.

Area 8. Reducing the negative consequences of drinking and alcohol intoxication

35. This target area includes policy options and interventions that focus directly on reducing the harm from alcohol intoxication and drinking without necessarily affecting the underlying alcohol consumption. Current evidence and good practices favour the complementary use of interventions within a broader strategy that prevents or reduces the negative consequences of drinking and alcohol intoxication. In implementing these approaches, managing the drinking environment or informing consumers, the perception of endorsing or promoting drinking should be avoided.

36. For this area **policy options and interventions** include:

(a) regulating the drinking context in order to minimize violence and disruptive behaviour, including serving alcohol in plastic containers or shatter-proof glass and management of alcohol-related issues at large-scale public events;

(b) enforcing laws against serving to intoxication and legal liability for consequences of harm resulting from intoxication caused by the serving of alcohol;

(c) enacting management policies relating to responsible serving of beverage on premises and training staff in relevant sectors in how better to prevent, identify and manage intoxicated and aggressive drinkers;

(d) reducing the alcoholic strength inside different beverage categories;

(e) providing necessary care or shelter for severely intoxicated people;

(f) providing consumer information about, and labelling alcoholic beverages to indicate, the harm related to alcohol.

Area 9. Reducing the public health impact of illicit alcohol and informally produced alcohol

37. Consumption of illicitly or informally produced alcohol could have additional negative health consequences due to a higher ethanol content and potential contamination with toxic substances, such as methanol. It may also hamper governments' abilities to tax and control legally produced alcohol. Actions to reduce these additional negative effects should be taken according to the prevalence of illicit and/or informal alcohol consumption and the associated harm. Good scientific, technical and institutional capacity should be in place for the planning and implementation of appropriate national, regional and international measures. Good market knowledge and insight into the composition and production of informal or illicit alcohol are also important, coupled with an appropriate legislative framework and active enforcement. These interventions should complement, not replace, other interventions to reduce harmful use of alcohol.

38. Production and sale of informal alcohol are ingrained in many cultures and are often informally controlled. Thus control measures could be different for illicit alcohol and informally produced alcohol and should be combined with awareness raising and community mobilization. Efforts to stimulate alternative sources of income are also important.

39. For this area **policy options and interventions** include:

(a) good quality control with regard to production and distribution of alcoholic beverages;

(b) regulating sales of informally produced alcohol and bringing it into the taxation system;

(c) an efficient control and enforcement system, including tax stamps;

(d) developing or strengthening tracking and tracing systems for illicit alcohol;

(e) ensuring necessary cooperation and exchange of relevant information on combating illicit alcohol among authorities at national and international levels;

(f) issuing relevant public warnings about contaminants and other health threats from informal or illicit alcohol.

Area 10. Monitoring and surveillance

40. Data from monitoring and surveillance create the basis for the success and appropriate delivery of the other nine policy options. Local, national and international monitoring and surveillance are needed in order to monitor the magnitude and trends of alcohol-related harms, to strengthen advocacy, to formulate policies and to assess impact of interventions. Monitoring should also capture the profile of people accessing services and the reason why people most affected are not accessing prevention and treatment services. Data may be available in other sectors, and good systems for coordination, information exchange and collaboration are necessary in order to collect the potentially broad range of information needed to have comprehensive monitoring and surveillance.

41. Development of sustainable national information systems using indicators, definitions and data-collection procedures compatible with WHO's global and regional information systems provides an important basis for effective evaluation of national efforts to reduce harmful use of alcohol and for monitoring trends at subregional, regional and global levels. Systematic continual collection, collation and analysis of data, timely dissemination of information and feedback to policy-makers and other stakeholders should be an integral part of implementation of any policy and intervention to reduce harmful use of alcohol. Collecting, analysing and disseminating information on harmful use of alcohol are resource-intensive activities.

42. For this area **policy options and interventions** include:

(a) establishing effective frameworks for monitoring and surveillance activities including periodic national surveys on alcohol consumption and alcohol-related harm and a plan for exchange and dissemination of information;

(b) establishing or designating an institution or other organizational entity responsible for collecting, collating, analysing and disseminating available data, including publishing national reports;

(c) defining and tracking a common set of indicators of harmful use of alcohol and of policy responses and interventions to prevent and reduce such use;

(d) creating a repository of data at the country level based on internationally agreed indicators and reporting data in the agreed format to WHO and other relevant international organizations;

(e) developing evaluation mechanisms with the collected data in order to determine the impact of policy measures, interventions and programmes put in place to reduce the harmful use of alcohol.

Global action: key role and components

43. Given the magnitude and the complexity of the problem, concerted global efforts must be in place to support Member States in the challenges they face at the national level. International coordination and collaboration create the synergies that are needed and provide increased leverage for Member States to implement evidence-based measures.

44. WHO, in cooperation with other organizations in the United Nations system and other international partners will:

(a) provide leadership;

(b) strengthen advocacy;

(c) formulate, in collaboration with Member States, evidence-based policy options;

(d) promote networking and exchange of experience among countries;

(e) strengthen partnerships and resource mobilization;

(f) coordinate monitoring of alcohol-related harm and the progress countries are making to address it.

45. Action by WHO and other international partners to support the implementation of the global strategy will be taken according to their mandates. International nongovernmental organizations, professional associations, research institutions and economic operators in the area of alcohol, all have important roles in enhancing the global action, as follows.

(a) Major partners within the United Nations system and intergovernmental organizations like ILO, UNICEF, WTO, UNDP, UNFPA, UNAIDS, United Nations Office on Drugs and Crime, and the World Bank group will be urged to increase collaboration and cooperation to prevent and reduce harmful use of alcohol, especially in developing and low- and middle-income countries.

(b) Civil society has an important role in warning about the impact of harmful use of alcohol on individuals, families and communities and in bringing additional commitment and resources for reducing alcohol-related harm. Nongovernmental organizations are especially encouraged to form wide networks and action groups to support the implementation of the global strategy.

(c) Research institutions and professional associations play a pivotal role in generating additional evidence for action and disseminating this to health professionals and the wider community. WHO collaborating centres have an important role in supporting the implementation and evaluation of the global strategy.

(d) Economic operators in alcohol production and trade are important players in their role as developers, producers, distributors, marketers and sellers of alcoholic beverages. They are especially encouraged to consider effective ways to prevent and reduce harmful use of alcohol within their core roles mentioned above, including self-regulatory actions and initiatives. They could also contribute by making available data on sales and consumption of alcohol beverages.

(e) The media play an increasingly important role, not only as a conveyer of news and information but also as a channel for commercial communications, and will be encouraged to support the intentions and activities of the global strategy.

Public health advocacy and partnership

46. International public health advocacy and partnership are needed for strengthened commitment and abilities of the governments and all relevant parties at all levels for reducing harmful use of alcohol worldwide.

47. WHO is committed to raising awareness of the public health problems caused by harmful use of alcohol and of the steps that can be taken to prevent and reduce such use in order to save lives and reduce suffering. WHO will engage with other international intergovernmental organizations and, as appropriate, international bodies representing key stakeholders, to ensure that relevant actors can contribute to reducing the harmful use of alcohol.

48. The Secretariat will provide support to Member States by:

(a) raising the awareness of the magnitude of public health problems caused by harmful use of alcohol and advocating for appropriate action at all levels to prevent and reduce such problems;

(b) advocating that attention is given to addressing the harmful use of alcohol in the agendas of relevant international and intergovernmental organizations in order to support policy coherence between health and other sectors at regional and global levels;

(c) promoting and facilitating international coordination, collaboration, partnerships and information exchange to ensure the needed synergies and concerted actions of all relevant parties;

(d) ensuring consistency, scientific soundness and clarity of key messages about preventing and reducing harmful use of alcohol;

(e) promoting intercountry networking and exchange of experiences;

(f) facilitating international networking in order to tackle specific and similar problems (for example, specific problems among indigenous or other minority groups or changing youth drinking cultures);

(g) advocating appropriate consideration by parties in international, regional and bilateral trade negotiations to the need and the ability of national and subnational governments to regulate alcohol distribution, sales and marketing, and thus to manage alcohol-related health and social costs;

(h) ensuring that the WHO Secretariat has processes in place to work with nongovernmental organizations and other civil society groups, taking into consideration any conflicts of interest that some nongovernmental organizations may have;

(i) continuing its dialogue with the private sector on how they best can contribute to the reduction of alcohol-related harm. Appropriate consideration will be given to the commercial interests involved and their possible conflict with public health objectives.

Technical support and capacity building

49. Many Member States need increased capacity and capability to create, enforce and sustain the necessary policy and legal frames and implementation mechanisms. Global action will support national action through the development of sustainable mechanisms and the provision of the necessary normative guidance and technical tools for effective technical support and capacity building, with particular focus on developing and low- and middle-income countries. Such actions must be in accordance with the national contexts, needs and priorities. Development of the necessary infrastructure for effective policy responses in countries with higher or increasing alcohol-attributable burden is an important prerequisite for attaining broader public health and developmental objectives.

50. WHO is committed to cooperate with other relevant actors at regional and global levels in order to provide technical guidance and support for strengthening institutional capacity to respond to public health problems caused by harmful use of alcohol. WHO will especially focus on support and building capacity in developing and low- and middle-income countries.

51. The Secretariat will provide support to Member States by:

(a) documenting and disseminating good models of health-service responses to alcohol-related problems;

(b) documenting and disseminating best practices and models of responses to alcohol-related problems in different sectors;

(c) drawing on expertise in other areas like road safety, taxation and justice with public health expertise in order to design effective models to prevent and reduce alcohol-related harm;

(d) providing normative guidance on effective and cost-effective prevention and treatment interventions in different settings;

(e) developing and strengthening global, regional and intercountry networks in order to help in sharing best practices and facilitating capacity building;

(f) responding to Member States' requests for support of their efforts to build the capacity to understand the implications of international trade and trade agreements for health.

Production and dissemination of knowledge

52. Important areas for global action will be monitoring trends in alcohol consumption, alcohol-attributable harm and the societal responses, analysing this information and facilitating timely dissemination. Available knowledge on the magnitude of harmful use of alcohol, and effectiveness and cost-effectiveness of preventive and treatment interventions should be further consolidated and expanded systematically at the global level, especially information on epidemiology of alcohol use and alcohol-related harm, impact of harmful use of alcohol on economic and social development and the spread of infectious diseases in developing and low- and middle-income countries.

53. The Global Information System on Alcohol and Health and its regional components were developed by WHO for dynamic presentation of the data on levels and patterns of alcohol consumption, alcohol-attributable health and social consequences and policy responses at all levels. Improving the global and regional data on alcohol and health requires development of national monitoring systems, regular reporting of data by designated focal points to WHO and strengthening the relevant surveillance activities.

54. WHO is committed to working with the relevant partners to shape the international research agenda on alcohol and health, build capacity for research and promote and support international research networks and projects to generate and disseminate data to inform policy and programme development.

55. The Secretariat will provide support to Member States by:

(a) providing an international clearinghouse for information on effective and cost-effective interventions to reduce harmful use of alcohol including promoting and facilitating exchange of information about effective treatment services;

(b) strengthening the Global Information System on Alcohol and Health and the comparative risk assessment of the alcohol-attributable disease burden;

(c) developing or refining appropriate data-collection mechanisms, based on comparable data and agreed indicators and definitions, in order to facilitate data collection, collation, analysis and dissemination at the global, regional and national levels;

(d) facilitating regional and global networks to support and complement national efforts, with a focus on knowledge production and information exchange;

(e) continuing its collaboration with international networks of scientists and health experts to promote research on various aspects of harmful use of alcohol;

(f) facilitating comparative effectiveness studies of different policy measures implemented in different cultural and developmental contexts;

(g) facilitating operational research to expand effective interventions and research on the relationship between harmful use of alcohol and social and health inequities.

Resource mobilization

56. The magnitude of alcohol-attributable disease and social burden is in sharp contradiction with the resources available at all levels to reduce harmful use of alcohol. Global development initiatives must take into account that developing and low- and middle-income countries need technical support – through aid and expertise – to establish and strengthen national policies and plans for the prevention of harmful use of alcohol and develop appropriate infrastructures, including those in health-care systems. Development agencies could consider reducing harmful use of alcohol as a priority area in developing and low- and middle-income countries with a high burden of disease attributable to harmful use of alcohol. Official development assistance provides opportunities to build sustainable institutional capacity in this area in developing and low- and middle-income countries, as do mechanisms for collaboration between developing countries. In that regard, Member States are urged to support each other in the implementation of the global strategy through international cooperation and financial assistance including official development assistance for developing countries.

57. WHO is committed to assist countries upon request in resource mobilization and pooling of available resources to support global and national action to reduce harmful use of alcohol in identified priority areas.

58. The Secretariat will provide support to Member States by:

(a) promoting exchange of experience and good practice in financing policies and interventions to reduce harmful use of alcohol;

(b) exploring new or innovative ways and means to secure adequate funding for implementation of the global strategy;

(c) collaborating with international partners, intergovernmental partners and donors to mobilize necessary resources to support developing and low- and middle-income countries in their efforts to reduce harmful use of alcohol.

Implementing the strategy

59. Successful implementation of the strategy will require concerted action by Member States, effective global governance and appropriate engagement of all relevant stakeholders. All actions listed in the strategy are proposed to support the achievement of the five objectives.

60. The Secretariat will report regularly on the global burden of alcohol-related harm, make evidence-based recommendations, and advocate action at all levels to prevent and reduce harmful use of alcohol. It will collaborate with other intergovernmental organizations and, as appropriate, other international bodies representing key stakeholders to ensure that action to reduce harmful use of alcohol receives appropriate priority and resources.

Links and interfaces with other strategies, plans and programmes

61. This global strategy builds upon regional initiatives such as the Framework for alcohol policy in the WHO European Region (resolution EUR/RC55/R1), the Regional strategy to reduce alcohol-related harm in the Western Pacific Region (resolution WPR/RC57. R5), Alcohol consumption control – policy options in the South-East Asia Region (resolution SEA/RC59/R8), Public health problems of alcohol consumption in the Eastern Mediterranean Region (resolution EM/RC53/R.5) and Actions to reduce the harmful use of alcohol in the African Region (document AFR/RC58/3).

62. Harmful use of alcohol is one of the four main risk factors highlighted in the action plan for the global strategy for the prevention and control of noncommunicable diseases (resolution WHA61.14). The strategy to reduce harmful use of alcohol builds on and links to the other risk factors for noncommunicable diseases and the disease-specific programmes, especially through the global strategy on diet, physical activity and health (resolution WHA57.17), tobacco control (resolution WHA56.1), health promotion and healthy lifestyle (resolution WHA57.16) and cancer prevention and control (resolution WHA58.22).

63. The strategy also links and aligns itself with other related activities in WHO, especially the Mental Health Gap Action Programme, including suicide prevention and management of other substance use disorders as well as programmatic activities on violence and health (resolution WHA56.24), road safety and health (resolution WHA57.10), child and adolescent health and development (resolution WHA56.21) and reproductive health (resolution WHA57.12).

64. With emerging evidence, greater attention is being given to the links between harmful use of alcohol and some infectious diseases and between harmful drinking and development. The strategy also links in with WHO's existing progammes on HIV/AIDS and tuberculosis and its work on reducing health inequities through action on the social determinants of health (resolution WHA62.14) and achieving the health-related development goals including those contained in the United Nations Millennium Declaration (resolution WHA58.30).

65. The implementation of a global strategy to reduce harmful use of alcohol provides a supportive framework for the WHO regional offices to formulate, revisit and implement region-specific policies and, together with the country offices, provide technical support to Member States. Emphasis will also be put on coordination within the Secretariat so that all actions relevant to harmful use of alcohol are in line with this strategy.

Monitoring progress and reporting mechanisms

66. For monitoring progress, the strategy requires appropriate mechanisms at different levels for assessment, reporting and re-programming. A framework with an impact-focused perspective is needed for assessing achievement of the strategy's objectives.

67. WHO's Global Survey on Alcohol and Health and the Global Information System on Alcohol and Health will be important parts of the reporting and monitoring mechanisms. The data-collecting tools of the latter will be adjusted to include the relevant reporting on the process and outcomes of implementation of the strategy at the national level.

68. Regular meetings of global and regional networks of national counterparts offer a mechanism for technical discussion of the implementation of the global strategy at different levels. In addition to taking stock of the process, these meetings could include detailed discussions of priority areas and topics relevant to implementation.

69. Reporting on the implementation of the global strategy to Member States will take place through regular reports to WHO regional committees and the Health Assembly. Information about implementation and progress should also be presented at regional or international forums and appropriate intergovernmental meetings.

RESOLUTION OF THE SIXTY-THIRD WORLD HEALTH ASSEMBLY (MAY 2010)
WHA63.13 GLOBAL STRATEGY TO REDUCE THE HARMFUL USE OF ALCOHOL

The Sixty-third World Health Assembly,

Having considered the report on strategies to reduce the harmful use of alcohol[1] and the draft global strategy annexed therein;

Recalling resolutions WHA58.26 on public-health problems caused by harmful use of alcohol and WHA61.4 on strategies to reduce the harmful use of alcohol;

1. **ENDORSES** the global strategy to reduce the harmful use of alcohol;

2. **AFFIRMS** that the global strategy to reduce the harmful use of alcohol aims to give guidance for action at all levels and to set priority areas for global action, and that it is a portfolio of policy options and measures that could be considered for implementation and adjusted as appropriate at the national level, taking into account national circumstances, such as religious and cultural contexts, national public health priorities, as well as resources, capacities and capabilities;

3. **URGES** Member States:[2]

    (1) to adopt and implement the global strategy to reduce the harmful use of alcohol as appropriate in order to complement and support public health policies in Member States to reduce the harmful use of alcohol, and to mobilize political will and financial resources for that purpose;

    (2) to continue implementation of the resolutions WHA61.4 on the strategies to reduce the harmful use of alcohol and WHA58.26 on public-health problems caused by harmful use of alcohol;

    (3) to ensure that implementation of the global strategy to reduce the harmful use of alcohol strengthens the national efforts to protect at-risk populations, young people and those affected by harmful drinking of others;

    (4) to ensure that implementation of the global strategy to reduce the harmful use of alcohol is reflected in the national monitoring systems and reported regularly to WHO's information system on alcohol and health;

---

1 Document A63/13.

2 And, where applicable, regional economic integration organizations.

4. REQUESTS the Director-General:

(1) to give sufficiently high organizational priority, and to assure adequate financial and human resources at all levels, to the prevention and reduction of harmful use of alcohol and implementation of the global strategy to reduce the harmful use of alcohol;

(2) to collaborate with and provide support to Member States, as appropriate, in implementing the global strategy to reduce the harmful use of alcohol and strengthening national responses to public health problems caused by the harmful use of alcohol;

(3) to monitor progress in implementing the global strategy to reduce the harmful use of alcohol and to report progress, through the Executive Board, to the Sixty-sixth World Health Assembly.

(Eighth plenary meeting, 21 May 2010 –
Committee A, fourth report)

ANNEX I
REPORT BY THE SECRETARIAT[1] TO THE SIXTY-THIRD WORLD HEALTH ASSEMBLY (MAY 2010)
STRATEGIES TO REDUCE THE HARMFUL USE OF ALCOHOL: DRAFT GLOBAL STRATEGY

1. In resolution WHA61.4 (Strategies to reduce the harmful use of alcohol) the Health Assembly requested the Director-General to submit to the Sixty-third World Health Assembly, through the Executive Board, a draft global strategy to reduce harmful use of alcohol. The Health Assembly urged Member States to collaborate with the Secretariat in developing a draft global strategy, and further requested the Director-General to collaborate and consult with Member States, as well as to consult with intergovernmental organizations, health professionals, nongovernmental organizations and economic operators on ways they could contribute to reducing harmful use of alcohol.

2. The Secretariat has drafted a strategy through an inclusive and broad collaborative process with Member States. In doing so, the Secretariat took into consideration the outcomes of consultations with other stakeholders on ways in which they can contribute to reducing the harmful use of alcohol. The draft strategy is based on existing best practices and available evidence of effectiveness and cost-effectiveness of strategies and interventions to reduce the harmful use of alcohol; this evidence is summarized in Annex II.

3. The consultative process started with a public, web-based hearing from 3 October to 15 November 2008, giving Member States and other stakeholders an opportunity to submit proposals on ways to reduce harmful use of alcohol. Two separate round-table discussions, one with nongovernmental organizations and health professionals and the other with economic operators, were organized in Geneva in November 2008 in order to collect views on ways these stakeholders could contribute to reducing harmful use of alcohol. Subsequently, a consultation with selected intergovernmental organizations was held (Geneva, 8 September 2009).[2]

4. The Secretariat began work on a draft strategy by preparing a discussion paper for further consultations with Member States. That paper was formulated on the basis of the deliberations of WHO's governing bodies and several regional committee sessions as well as the similar outcomes of those bodies pertaining to other related areas such as noncommunicable diseases, mental health, violence and injury prevention, cancer, family and community health, social determinants of health, HIV/AIDS, and trade and health. Its content was also influenced by the outcomes of the Secretariat's technical activities on alcohol and health, including the relevant meetings of technical experts. The discussion paper was sent to the Member States and posted on the WHO web site.

---

1 Originally presented as document A63/13.

2 See the WHO web site for further information about the process of implementing resolution WHA61.4 and links to the various documents referred to in this report: http://www.who.int/substance_abuse/activities/globalstrategy/en/index.html.

5. Six regional technical consultations were held between February and May 2009, attended by participants nominated by governments of 149 Member States. Three consultations were held in the WHO Regional Offices for Africa, Europe and the Eastern Mediterranean. The governments of Brazil, Thailand and New Zealand, respectively, hosted the consultations for Member States in the Region of the Americas and the South-East Asia and Western Pacific regions. In all these regional consultations, Member States were invited to provide their views on the possible areas for global action and coordination outlined in the discussion paper, and on how the strategy could best take into account national needs and priorities. In addition, Member States were encouraged to provide information on current national and subregional processes that could contribute to the strategy development process, as well as examples of best practices, with special emphasis on at-risk populations, young people and those affected by the harmful drinking of others.

6. In preparing a working document for developing a draft global strategy to reduce harmful use of alcohol the Secretariat built on the outcomes of the regional consultations with Member States and took into consideration the outcomes of the previous consultative process with all stakeholders on ways in which they could contribute to reducing the harmful use of alcohol. The resulting document provided background information and suggested aims, objectives and guiding principles for a global strategy, target areas and a set of policy measures and interventions that it was proposed Member States could implement at the national level. The working document was sent to Member States in August 2009 with an invitation for written feedback on its content, and posted on the WHO web site. The Secretariat received written feedback from 40 Member States.

7. To continue the collaboration with Member States on the draft strategy the Secretariat held an informal consultation with Member States on 8 October 2009 in Geneva in order to discuss the feedback on the working document and to offer an opportunity for Member States to provide further guidance on finalizing a draft global strategy. Further taking into account the outcome of that informal consultation, the Secretariat finalized a draft global strategy.

8. In January 2010, at its 126th session,[1] the Executive Board considered an earlier version of this report and the draft strategy. During the session, discussions on the draft global strategy were also held in an open-ended informal working group, co-chaired by Cuba and Sweden. Consensus was reached on a revised text. The Board adopted resolution EB126.R11 in which it recommends the Health Assembly to endorse the global strategy.

Action by the Health Assembly

9. The Health Assembly is invited to adopt the resolution recommended by the Executive Board contained in resolution EB126.R11.

---

1 See document EB126/2010/REC/2 , summary record of the eleventh meeting.

ANNEX II
EVIDENCE FOR THE EFFECTIVENESS AND COST-EFFECTIVENESS OF INTERVENTIONS TO REDUCE HARMFUL USE OF ALCOHOL

1. During recent years a substantial body of knowledge has accumulated on feasibility, effectiveness and cost-effectiveness of different policy options and interventions aimed at reducing the harmful use of alcohol. Most of the evidence comes from high-income countries, but the number of studies in low- and middle-income countries is steadily increasing. This annex briefly summarizes the main findings of research that can inform policy and programme development to prevent and reduce harmful use of alcohol.

2. There are many reasons for placing an emphasis on education and information, including the notion that a population should know about and understand harmful alcohol use and associated health risks, even though the evidence base indicates that the impact of alcohol-education programmes on harmful use of alcohol is small. To be effective, education about alcohol needs to go beyond providing information about the risks of harmful use of alcohol to promoting the availability of effective interventions and mobilizing public opinion and support for effective alcohol policies.

3. The evidence for the effectiveness of early identification and brief advice for persons with hazardous and harmful alcohol use is extensive and comes from a large number of systematic reviews from a variety of health-care settings in different countries. The findings show that more intensive advice appears to be no more effective than less intensive advice. Cognitive-behavioural therapies and pharmacological therapies do have a positive effect in treatment of alcohol dependence and related problems. Consideration should also be given to integrated treatment for co-morbid conditions, such as for hypertension, tuberculosis and HIV/AIDS, and to self-help groups.

4. An important component of community action programmes, which has been shown to change young people's drinking behaviour and on alcohol-related harm such as traffic crashes and violence, is media advocacy. Another approach to community action in low-income countries has been to encourage communities to mobilize public opinion to address local determinants of increased levels of harmful use of alcohol.

5. Strong evidence supports the conclusion that a sufficiently low limit for blood alcohol concentration (0.02% to 0.05%) is effective in reducing drink-driving casualties. Both intensive random breath-testing, whereby police regularly stop drivers on a random basis to check their blood alcohol concentrations, and selective breath-testing, where vehicles are stopped and drivers suspected of drink-driving are breath-tested, reduce alcohol-related injuries and fatalities. There is evidence for some effectiveness of setting lower limits for blood alcohol concentrations (including a zero level) for young or novice drivers, administrative suspension of the driver's licence in case of a

56688

blood alcohol concentration above the limit, mandatory counselling or treatment for alcohol-related conditions and the use of an ignition interlock for repeat drink drivers. Consistent enforcement by police with random or selective breath-testing followed by effective sanctions is essential and should be supported by sustained publicity and awareness campaigns.

6. Evidence from a range of settings demonstrates the importance of a legal framework for reducing the physical availability of alcohol that encompasses restrictions on both the sale and serving of alcohol. Having a licensing system for the sale of alcohol allows for the opportunity for control, since infringement of laws can be met by revocation of the licence. Implementation of laws that set a minimum age for the purchase of alcohol show clear reductions in drinking-driving casualties and other alcohol-related harm; the most effective means of enforcement is on sellers, who have a business interest in retaining the right to sell alcohol. An increased density of alcohol outlets is associated with increased levels of alcohol consumption among young people, increased levels of assault, and other harm such as homicide, child abuse and neglect, self-inflicted injury, and, with less consistent evidence, road traffic injuries. Reducing the hours or days of sale of alcoholic beverages leads to fewer alcohol-related problems, including homicides and assaults.

7. A growing volume of evidence from longitudinal youth studies points to an impact of various forms of alcohol marketing on initiation of youth drinking and riskier patterns of youth drinking. Some results remain contested, in part owing to methodological difficulties. To be effective, systems to regulate marketing need sufficient incentives to succeed; in general, regulatory frameworks are most active where pressure from the government is greatest, and can only work as long as there is provision for third-party review of complaints about violations. Sanctions and the threat of sanctions are needed to ensure compliance.

8. The more affordable alcohol is – the lower its price, or the more disposable income people have – the more it is consumed and the greater the level of related harm in both high- and low-income countries. Modelling shows that setting a minimum price per unit gram of alcohol reduces consumption and alcohol-related harm. Both price increases and setting a minimum price are estimated to have a much greater impact on drinkers who consume more than on those who consume less. Natural experiments consequent to economic treaties have shown that, as alcohol taxes and prices were lowered to offset cross-border trade, so sales, alcohol consumption and alcohol-related harm have usually increased.

9. Some evidence indicates that safety-oriented design of the premises where alcoholic beverages are served and the employment of security staff, in part to reduce potential violence, can reduce alcohol-related harm. Even though interventions modifying the behaviour of those serving alcohol appear ineffective on their own, they may be effective when backed up by enforcement by police or liquor-licence inspectors. Harm-reduction approach can be supported by stronger promotion of products with a lower alcohol concentration, together with mandated health warnings on alcohol-product containers. Although such warnings do not lead to changes in drinking behaviour, they do impact on intentions to change drinking patterns and remind consumers about the risks associated with alcohol consumption.

10. Good scientific, technical and institutional capacity should be in place for the planning and implementation of appropriate national, regional and international measures. Good market knowledge and insight into the composition and production of informal or illicit alcohol are also important, coupled with an appropriate legislative framework and active enforcement. Control measures should be combined with awareness raising and community mobilization.

11. A bibliography of the main sources of evidence will be made available on the WHO web site.[1]

---

1 http://www.who.int/substance_abuse/activities/globalstrategy/en/index.html (accessed 20 November 2009).

ANNEX III
RESOLUTION OF THE SIXTY-FIRST WORLD HEALTH ASSEMBLY (MAY 2008)
WHA61.14 STRATEGIES TO REDUCE THE HARMFUL USE OF ALCOHOL

The Sixty-first World Health Assembly,

Having considered the report on strategies to reduce the harmful use of alcohol[1] and the further guidance on strategies and policy element options therein;

Reaffirming resolutions WHA32.40 on development of the WHO programme on alcohol-related problems, WHA36.12 on alcohol consumption and alcohol-related problems, development of national policies and programmes, WHA42.20 on prevention and control of drug and alcohol abuse and WHA57.16 on health promotion and healthy lifestyles;

Recalling resolution WHA58.26 on public-health problems caused by harmful use of alcohol and decision WHA60(10);

Noting the report by the Secretariat presented to the Sixtieth World Health Assembly on evidence-based strategies and interventions to reduce alcohol-related harm, including the addendum on a global assessment of public health problems caused by harmful use of alcohol;[2]

Noting the second report of the WHO Expert Committee on Problems Related to Alcohol Consumption[3] and acknowledging that effective strategies and interventions that target the general population, vulnerable groups, individuals and specific problems are available and should be optimally combined in order to reduce alcohol-related harm;

Mindful that such strategies and interventions must be implemented in a way that takes into account different national, religious and cultural contexts, including national public health problems, needs and priorities, and differences in Member States' resources, capacities and capabilities;

Deeply concerned by the extent of public health problems associated with harmful use of alcohol, including injuries and violence, and possible links to certain communicable diseases, thereby adding to the disease burden, in both developing and developed countries;

Mindful that international cooperation in reducing public health problems caused by the harmful use of alcohol is intensifying, and of the need to mobilize the necessary support at global and regional levels,

---

1 Document A61/13.

2 Documents A60/14 and A60/14 Add.1.

3 WHO Technical Report Series, No. 944, 2007.

1. **URGES** Member States:

    (1) to collaborate with the Secretariat in developing a draft global strategy on harmful use of alcohol based on all evidence and best practices, in order to support and complement public health policies in Member States, with special emphasis on an integrated approach to protect at-risk populations, young people and those affected by harmful drinking of others;

    (2) to develop, in interaction with relevant stakeholders, national systems for monitoring alcohol consumption, its health and social consequences and the policy responses, and to report regularly to WHO's regional and global information systems;

    (3) to consider strengthening national responses, as appropriate and where necessary, to public health problems caused by harmful use of alcohol, on the basis of evidence on effectiveness and cost-effectiveness of strategies and interventions to reduce alcohol-related harm generated in different contexts;

2. **REQUESTS** the Director-General:

    (1) to prepare a draft global strategy to reduce harmful use of alcohol that is based on all available evidence and existing best practices and that addresses relevant policy options, taking into account different national, religious and cultural contexts, including national public health problems, needs and priorities, and differences in Member States' resources, capacities and capabilities;

    (2) to ensure that the draft global strategy will include a set of proposed measures recommended for States to implement at the national level, taking into account the national circumstances of each country;

    (3) to include full details of ongoing and emerging regional, subregional and national processes as vital contributions to a global strategy;

    (4) to collaborate and consult with Member States, as well as consult with intergovernmental organizations, health professionals, nongovernmental organizations and economic operators on ways they could contribute to reducing harmful use of alcohol;

    (5) to submit to the Sixty-third World Health Assembly, through the Executive Board, a draft global strategy to reduce harmful use of alcohol.

(Eighth plenary meeting, 24 May 2008 –
Committee A, second report)

ANNEX IV
RESOLUTION OF THE FIFTY-EIGHT WORLD HEALTH ASSEMBLY (MAY 2005)
WHA58.26 PUBLIC-HEALTH PROBLEMS CAUSED BY HARMFUL USE OF ALCOHOL

The Fifty-eighth World Health Assembly,

Having considered the report on public health problems caused by harmful use of alcohol;[1]

Reaffirming resolutions WHA32.40 on development of the WHO programme on alcohol-related problems, WHA36.12 on alcohol consumption and alcohol-related problems: development of national policies and programmes, WHA42.20 on prevention and control of drug and alcohol abuse, WHA55.10 on mental health: responding to the call for action, WHA57.10 on road safety and health, WHA57.16 on health promotion and healthy lifestyles, and WHA57.17 on the Global Strategy on Diet, Physical Activity and Health;

Recalling *The world health report 2002*, which indicated that 4% of the burden of disease and 3.2% of all deaths globally were attributed to alcohol, and that alcohol was the foremost risk to health in low-mortality developing countries and the third in developed countries;[2]

Recognizing that the patterns, context and overall level of alcohol consumption influence the health of the population as a whole, and that harmful drinking is among the foremost underlying causes of disease, injury, violence – especially domestic violence against women and children – disability, social problems and premature deaths, is associated with mental ill-health, has a serious impact on human welfare affecting individuals, families, communities and society as a whole, and contributes to social and health inequalities;

Emphasizing the risk of harm due to alcohol consumption, particularly in the context of driving a vehicle, at the workplace, and during pregnancy;

Alarmed by the extent of public health problems associated with harmful consumption of alcohol and the trends in hazardous drinking, particularly among young people, in many Member States;

Recognizing that intoxication with alcohol is associated with high-risk behaviours, including the use of other psychoactive substances and unsafe sex;

Concerned about the economic loss to society resulting from harmful alcohol consumption, including costs to the health, social welfare and criminal justice systems, lost productivity, and reduced economic development;

Recognizing the threats posed to public health by the factors that have given rise to increasing availability and accessibility of alcoholic beverages in some Member States;

---

1 Document A58/18.

2 *The world health report 2002. Reducing risks, promoting healthy life.* Geneva, World Health Organization, 2002.

Noting the growing body of evidence of the effectiveness of strategies and measures aimed at reducing alcohol-related harm;

Mindful that individuals should be empowered to make positive, life-changing decisions for themselves on matters such as consumption of alcohol;

Taking due consideration of the religious and cultural sensitivities of a considerable number of Member States with regard to consumption of alcohol, and emphasizing that use of the word "harmful" in this resolution refers only to public-health effects of alcohol consumption, without prejudice to religious beliefs and cultural norms in any way,

1. REQUESTS Member States:

   (1) to develop, implement and evaluate effective strategies and programmes for reducing the negative health and social consequences of harmful use of alcohol;

   (2) to encourage mobilization and active and appropriate engagement of all concerned social and economic groups, including scientific, professional, nongovernmental and voluntary bodies, the private sector, civil society and industry associations, in reducing harmful use of alcohol;

   (3) to support the work requested of the Director-General below, including, if necessary, through voluntary contributions by interested Member States;

2. REQUESTS the Director-General:

   (1) to strengthen the Secretariat's capacity to provide support to Member States in monitoring alcohol-related harm and to reinforce the scientific and empirical evidence of effectiveness of policies;

   (2) to consider intensifying international cooperation in reducing public-health problems caused by the harmful use of alcohol, and to mobilize the necessary support at global and regional levels;

   (3) to consider also conducting further scientific studies pertaining to different aspects of possible impact of alcohol consumption on public health;

   (4) to report to the Sixtieth World Health Assembly on evidence-based strategies and interventions to reduce alcohol-related harm, including a comprehensive assessment of public-health problems caused by harmful use of alcohol

   (5) to draw up recommendations for effective policies and interventions to reduce alcohol-related harm, and to develop technical tools that will support Member States in implementing and evaluating recommended strategies and programmes;

   (6) to strengthen global and regional information systems through further collection and analysis of data on alcohol consumption and its health and social consequences, providing technical support to Member States and promoting research where such data are not available;

(7)   to promote and support global and regional activities aimed at identifying and managing alcohol-use disorders in health-care settings and enhancing the capacity of health-care professionals to address problems of their patients associated with harmful patterns of alcohol consumption;

(8)   to collaborate with Member States, intergovernmental organizations, health professionals, nongovernmental organizations and other relevant stakeholders to promote the implementation of effective policies and programmes to reduce harmful alcohol consumption;

(9)   to organize open consultations with representatives of the industry, agriculture and trade sectors in order to limit the health impact of harmful alcohol consumption;

(10) to report through the Executive Board to the Sixtieth World Health Assembly on progress made in implementation of this resolution.

(Ninth plenary meeting, 25 May 2005 –
Committee B, fourth report)